"Sweat, Swear & Succeed: The Hilarious Path to Weight Loss and Diabetes Control.
"

by Nikole de La Mer

I'll never forget when at age 47 I was diagnosed with diabetes three years before that I was diagnosed with fight or flight syndrome and I had no idea how deeply they were entwined.No matter what I did, no matter what I tried, my blood sugar remained high and my weight remained higher. After a lot of research and a little bit of trial and error and a shit load of luck I discovered the link between stress diabetes and fight or flight syndrome and that changed everything.

I tried keto I tried the Mediterranean diet I tried every new fad or breakthrough in weight loss there was and nothing changed I was still heavy and my blood sugar was creeping up more and more every day.

Until one day I put my money where my mouth is and I started taking good care of myself spiritually physically mentally and socially. I woke up every morning and developed a morning routine that I did no matter what or where I was rain or shine and it made a huge difference I also stopped worrying so much about how much I eat and about what I eat and decided to choose real food.

So I hope you enjoyed this book which is inspired of course by my own journey and written in my style of humor swearing and science. These techniques helped me go from a sorry size 22 to a happy size 16. And still going.

Carry on my stressed out babes….. And enjoy. Go on, read all ready.

So here we are again, we need to stop meeting like this, or do we?

Before you can start the process one of the things you need to know is what does my fat do for me?

Sounds like a stupid question, and I was right there with you when the idea was broached to me. What does my fat do for me? Well it keeps me fucking unhealthy, unhappy and visually unappealing I thought, but here's a great big truth bomb: your fat has given you a benefit or you wouldn't have it. Diabetes is a disease of the pancreas, not the mouth and fight or flight Syndrome comes from constant stress and trauma. No where does it say you have to be fat to be traumatized or diabetic. Period.

SO take a few moments to ask yourself: what does fat do for me? Does it protect me from bad experiences or people? Does food make me feel loved and cared about? Or does your fat make you feel nurtured and comforted? It is always one of those three. Ain't life a bitch? A bad childhood, or major trauma are what's keeping you fat and not happy.

Once you determine which of those it is, do some therapy, tapping, journaling surrounding it and start finding other ways to replace fat. Like pedicures, reading, a good friend or flowers and be your own mother, best friend, dessert or safety net. Cuz you are so worth it babe! Truly beautiful and a work of art. Trust me.

Chapter 1: The Weighty Issue of Diabetes

Ladies, gather 'round, because we're about to dive headfirst into the wild and wacky world of diabetes and weight loss. Yeah, I know, it's not the glamorous vacation destination you had in mind, but trust me, there's an adventure in here that's worth every calorie counted and every drop of sweat shed.

Diabetes: The Unwanted Intruder

Let's talk about diabetes. It's that uninvited guest who shows up to your party and refuses to leave, like that annoying neighbor who always borrows your lawnmower and never returns it. You didn't ask for it, but here it is, messing with your life like a bull in a China shop.

Now, before you start sulking, let me be clear: diabetes is not a death sentence. It's more like a challenging puzzle. Imagine someone handed you a Rubik's Cube set to expert mode – that's diabetes. It's complicated, frustrating, but totally conquerable with the right moves.

The Extra Weight Conundrum

Now, let's talk about the elephant in the room – or should I say, the extra weight in the room? Carrying around those extra pounds is like giving diabetes a backstage pass to your blood sugar concert. It's like saying, "Hey, come on in and mess things up!"

I know what you're thinking hey Nicole if I could lose the weight I fucking would don't you think I've tried that already? And I know exactly how you feel. Using

You see, excess weight messes with your body's insulin response – that's the hormone responsible for keeping your blood sugar in check. It's like your body's cells have decided to go on strike, refusing to listen to insulin's commands. Result? Your blood sugar levels go haywire, and you're left scratching your head. The higher your blood sugar is the easier it is to lose weight but that's not a good way to lose weight it means you're not getting the nutrition you need but the lower your insulin is the more weight you put on or the harder it is for you to lose what you have so it's just a vicious fucking circle. Making it a frustrating ride on the worlds worst roller coaster.

But here's the silver lining: losing even a little weight can be like putting insulin back in the driver's seat. It's like saying, "Okay, buddy, you're in charge again." Your blood sugar levels start to behave, and you get back some control over your own body.

The Cliffhanger: What Lies Ahead?

Alright, enough of the heavy stuff. It's time to lighten the mood and crack a few jokes because this journey is going to be a blender of emotions, sweat, and the occasional swear word. But don't worry; we're in it together, and we're going to come out on top.

In the upcoming chapters, we're going to tackle nutrition with the elegance of a ballerina, hit the gym with the gusto of a Viking warrior, and face down stress like a Zen master with a sense of humor. Oh yes, humor is going to be our secret weapon, and the occasional colorful word. Well, consider that our battle cry.

So, strap in, ladies, because this adventure has just begun, and it's going to be a hell of a ride. We're setting out on a quest filled with sweat, swearing, and, most importantly, success. Grab your determination and your sense of humor, because we're marching forward, and the best is yet to come.

Chapter 2: Diabetes & the Fight or Flight Fiasco

Alright, ladies, let's get down to the nitty-gritty of diabetes and this whole fight or flight fiasco. We're about to dive into the science of stress, diabetes, and why our bodies sometimes feel like they're in the middle of a rollercoaster ride without the safety harness.

The Fight or Flight Circus

So, what exactly is this "fight or flight" thing, and why does it have anything to do with diabetes? Well, imagine you're a cavewoman, and you stumble upon a saber-toothed tiger. Your body goes into overdrive mode – heart pounding, muscles tensing, and senses on high alert. That's your fight or flight response, a survival mechanism.

Fast forward to today, and our modern lives are like one big stress-fest. It might not be tigers we're dealing with, but it's deadlines, traffic jams, and an inbox that won't quit. Our bodies, however, haven't quite caught up with the times. They're still stuck in cavewoman mode, thinking that a traffic jam is a life-or-death situation.

Cortisol: The Stress Hormone We Love to Hate

Meet cortisol – your body's stress hormone. When the fight or flight response kicks in, cortisol is like the orchestra conductor, waving its baton and making everything more dramatic. It's essential for survival, but too much of it can lead to all sorts of mischief.

Now, here's where diabetes enters the scene, like an unwanted guest crashing a party. Cortisol has a knack for messing with your blood sugar levels. It's like it has a hotline to diabetes, and they're having a little secret chat behind your back. Cortisol whispers, "Hey, let's raise blood sugar levels," and diabetes nods in agreement.

The result? Your blood sugar levels go on a rollercoaster ride of their own, leaving you feeling like you're stuck in a never-ending episode of a soap opera. You're up, you're down, and you're left wondering, "What the hell is going on?"

The Cliffhanger: Taming the Beast

So, here's the deal, ladies. Diabetes, the fight or flight response, and excess weight are like the three musketeers, only without the fancy swords and heroic deeds. They're conspiring against you, and its high time we show them who's boss. Slip[on the mental latex corset, and lets make Diabetes our bitch.

In the chapters to come, we're going to explore ways to outsmart cortisol, kick diabetes in the rear, and make that excess weight wish it never showed up to the party. But remember, we're not just here to survive; we're here to thrive.

So, gear up, because we're about to conquer this fight or flight fiasco with humor as our shield and knowledge as our sword. We'll emerge from this battle stronger, wittier, and with a blood sugar chart that finally makes sense. The journey ahead may be challenging, but it's also going to be a hell of a good time. So, stay tuned, my fierce warriors, because the best is yet to come.

Chapter 3: Eating Smart, Not Less

Alright, ladies, grab your forks and your witty banter because we're about to tackle one of the most crucial aspects of managing diabetes while shedding those stubborn pounds: eating smart, not less.

The Dieting Dilemma

Let's face it; the word "diet" has become the Voldemort of our lives. It's become synonymous with deprivation, misery, and the endless battle of willpower. But here's the thing: we're not about deprivation here; we're about empowerment. It's time to redefine what "diet" means for us.

Diabetes may have brought us to this crossroads, but we're not backing down. It's time to put on our culinary armor and wade into battle with knowledge as our sword.

The Power of Portion Control

Alright, let's start with the basics: portion control. Now, I know it sounds about as exciting as watching paint dry, but bear with me. Portion control is like the Jedi mind trick of weight management. It allows you to enjoy your favorite foods without your blood sugar spiraling into chaos.

So, how do we do it? Well, we can use our good old hands as guides. Your palm represents your protein portion, your closed fist is for veggies, your thumb is for fats, and your cupped hand is for carbs. It's like having your very own portion control toolkit at your fingertips.

Now, I can already hear some of you groaning, "But I'll be hungry!" Fear not, my friend, because we're not just reducing portions; we're also boosting the quality of what we eat.

The Mighty Micronutrients

Micronutrients might sound like something straight out of a sci-fi movie, but they're the unsung heroes of a healthy diet. These are the vitamins and minerals that keep our bodies ticking like finely tuned machines.

Let's talk about fiber. It's like the magical broomstick that sweeps away those pesky blood sugar spikes. You'll find fiber in foods like whole grains, fruits, and veggies. It not only keeps your blood sugar steady but also leaves you feeling full and satisfied.

Then there's protein, our trusty sidekick in the battle against hunger. Protein helps keep those cravings at bay and is essential for maintaining lean muscle mass – something we absolutely want in our corner when fighting the weight loss war.

And don't forget fats – the good ones, that is. Avocado, nuts, and olive oil are like the superheroes of fats. They keep your heart happy, and your taste buds satisfied.

The Label Decoder

Okay, let's talk about something we all love to hate – reading food labels. It's like deciphering an ancient scroll, but fear not, because I've got some tricks up my sleeve to make it less painful.

First, check out the serving size. Sometimes what looks like a single portion is enough to feed a small army.

Next, peek at the total carbs and the fiber content. Subtract the fiber from the total carbs to find the "net carbs." These are the ones that have the biggest impact on your blood sugar.

And don't forget about sugar. It hides under all sorts of aliases – glucose, fructose, corn syrup, you name it. Keep an eye out for these sneaky sugars that can send your blood sugar on a rollercoaster ride.

Eating Out with Style

Now, I know life isn't always about home-cooked meals. We love to dine out, socialize, and indulge in the pleasures of restaurant cuisine. But dining out doesn't mean diabetes and weight loss are taking the night off.

When you're at a restaurant, don't be afraid to customize your order. Ask for dressings and sauces on the side, opt for grilled instead of fried, and choose whole grains when available. You're the boss of your meal, and you can make it work for you.

The Cliffhanger: What's Cooking?

So, there you have it, ladies – a crash course in eating smart, not less. We've learned about portion control, the power of micronutrients, and how to decode those tricky food labels. We've even discovered that dining out can be a breeze with the right approach.

But don't rest your culinary swords just yet, because the kitchen adventures are only beginning. In the chapters ahead, we'll delve into meal planning, recipes that will make your taste buds sing, and strategies for eating mindfully without feeling like you're missing out on life.

Stay tuned, because the feast is just getting started, and we're about to cook up a storm – with a side of humor, of course. So, sharpen those knives, and let's get ready to conquer the kitchen, one delicious meal at a time.

Ladies, we're back in the kitchen, and it's time to roll up our sleeves and dive deeper into the delicious world of eating smart, not less.

Mastering Meal Planning

Meal planning might sound as exciting as watching paint dry, but it's the secret weapon in your culinary arsenal. It's like having a game plan for a championship match – it sets you up for success.

Start by looking at your week ahead. Are you facing a busy workweek? Social events? Family dinners? Knowing what's on the horizon helps you plan meals that suit your schedule and your diabetes management goals.

Make a menu and a shopping list. This not only saves you time but also helps you make healthier choices. Stick to your list like it's a treasure map and avoid the temptation to stray into the snack aisle.

Recipes That Rock

Now, let's talk about recipes. We want meals that are not only good for our blood sugar but also taste like they're straight out of a five-star restaurant.

Think of your plate as a canvas waiting to be painted with color, flavor, and excitement. Experiment with herbs and spices to add pizzazz to your dishes. Lemon zest, garlic, ginger, and a sprinkle of chili flakes can turn a plain chicken breast into a culinary masterpiece.

And don't forget the magic of meal prepping. Spend a Sunday afternoon in the kitchen, preparing batches of your favorite dishes. Portion them out, and you've got grab-and-go meals for the week ahead. It's like having your own personal chef!

Mindful Eating: Savor Every Bite

Eating mindfully isn't about chewing each bite fifty times (unless that's your thing). It's about savoring your food, being present at mealtime, and listening to your body.

Start by putting away distractions – no TV, no smartphone scrolling. Focus on your meal and savor every bite. This not only makes the meal more enjoyable but also helps you recognize when you're satisfied.

Mindful eating is like the art of the ninja. It helps you dodge those mindless munching moments when you're not even hungry. So, take your time, chew slowly, and enjoy the symphony of flavors in every bite.

Dining Out: The Social Culinary Ballet

Eating at a restaurant can be like performing a culinary ballet, and you're the lead dancer. But don't let the fancy menus intimidate you; you're the boss of your meal.

Start by scanning the menu for keywords like "grilled," "baked," or "steamed." These are your allies in the battle against hidden fats and extra calories.

Don't be shy about asking your server questions. They're like the tour guides of your dining experience. Inquire about ingredient substitutions, portion sizes, and preparation methods. A simple request can make your meal diabetes-friendly without sacrificing flavor.

The Cliffhanger: Ready, Set, Cook!

So, there you have it, ladies – a hearty helping of knowledge and strategies for eating smart, not less. We've mastered meal planning, explored the magic of recipes, and learned the art of mindful eating and dining out like culinary ninjas.

But the kitchen adventures are far from over. In the chapters that follow, we'll delve into specific meal ideas, explore creative substitutions, and even tackle those inevitable moments when cravings strike. The culinary journey ahead is filled with flavor, fun, and a healthy dose of humor.

The thing to remember, is have fun. No really have fun! Choose the amount of carbs to enjoy in a day, and design a bad ass meal plan around it. For instance, I keep my carbs under 200 a day and usually aim for 150. 3 meals and 2 snacks. Also, remember top has protein with everything. Everything. Like a bunch of peanuts before chocolate cake, kind of everything. Did I say chocolate cake? Why yes, yes I did. Don't deprive yourself, maintain yourself baby. That's the key to everything.

Have fun, watch your portions and stay within your carb ration you beautiful badass bitch…so get cooking already!

Chapter 4: Exercise: From Couch Potato to Powerhouse

Alright, my fellow diabetes warriors, it's time to get moving! We're diving headfirst into the world of exercise, where sweat is our battle paint, and our goal is to transform from couch potatoes into powerhouse superwomen.

Why Traditional Exercise Won't Cut It

Now, you might be thinking, "Exercise? That's the easy part, right?" Well, not quite. You see, diabetes and its sidekicks, fight or flight syndrome and extra weight, have made the exercise game a bit trickier for us. But don't worry; we're up for the challenge.

Let's address the elephant in the room – traditional exercise. You know the drill: hours on a treadmill, endless reps of exercises that make you feel like a hamster on a wheel, and the dreaded burpees that could make even a drill sergeant cringe. But guess what? Traditional exercise isn't always our best friend when we're battling diabetes and its companions.

The Problem with the Dreaded Blood Sugar Rollercoaster

Traditional exercise can send our blood sugar levels on a wild rollercoaster ride, and not the fun kind. It can cause your blood sugar to plummet to the floor, leaving you shaky and hangry. Or it can spike to the heavens, making you feel like you're about to take off on a sugar rocket.

Why does this happen? Well, when you exercise, your muscles are like hungry little monsters, gobbling up glucose for energy. That's great, but sometimes they get a little too greedy, and they don't listen when insulin tries to keep things in check.

And let's not forget our friend, fight or flight syndrome. When stress hormones like cortisol are in the mix, they can send your blood sugar on a rollercoaster ride of their own. It's like they're playing a cruel joke on you.

Enter: Smart Exercise Strategies

Now that we've exposed the flaws in traditional exercise, let's talk about how we can outsmart this blood sugar rollercoaster. It's time to embrace exercise in a way that works for us – diabetes, fight or flight syndrome, and all.

The Power of Strength Training

Strength training is like the superhero of the exercise world, especially for women dealing with diabetes. No need to pump iron,, go for the superhero resistance training. It helps build lean muscle mass, which is your secret weapon against blood sugar spikes.

Muscles are like little glucose sponges. When you engage in strength training, your muscles become more insulin sensitive, meaning they're better at listening to insulin and regulating your blood sugar. It's like having an army of blood sugar bouncers, making sure things stay in order.

Now, I'm not talking about pumping iron like a bodybuilder (unless that's your thing, then go for it!). Even light resistance exercises with resistance bands or bodyweight exercises can do wonders for your blood sugar control.

The Art of Cardio: Low and Slow

Cardio exercise, like jogging or spinning, can be a powerful tool, but we need to approach it with a strategy. Instead of going full throttle, opt for a low and slow approach.

Short, moderate-intensity workouts are our friends. These 20 minute miracles can help improve insulin sensitivity and keep that blood sugar rollercoaster in check. Brisk walking, swimming, or even dancing around your living room to your favorite tunes are great options. Make sure you add calming yoga to your daily routine. Not the acrobatic shit that ties you up like a pretzel, more like restorative or Yin yoga for the win.

Timing Is Everything

When it comes to exercise, timing is everything, especially when you're dealing with diabetes and fight or flight syndrome. You don't want to send your blood sugar plummeting into the abyss during your workout.

Aim to exercise about 10 minutes after a meal. This allows your body to have a steady supply of glucose for energy, reducing the risk of a blood sugar crash, and makes your muscles more sensitive to insulin. Stoll it out baby. Take a nice 10 minute walk after a meal or if weather is not walk friendly dance a little after a meal. Nothing like dinner and dancing to make a girl happy and healthy.

If you prefer to exercise in a fasted state, go for a short, gentle workout, like a leisurely walk. And always, always have a snack nearby in case you start to feel those dreaded low blood sugar symptoms.

The Cliffhanger: Unleashing Our Inner Powerhouses

So, there you have it, ladies – the lowdown on exercise and why traditional methods might not be our best friends right now. We've uncovered the flaws in the blood sugar rollercoaster and discovered that strength training and low-intensity cardio are our secret weapons.

But we're not done yet. In the chapters ahead, we'll explore ways to stay active, and strategies to make exercise a part of your daily routine. It's time to unleash our inner powerhouses and conquer the world – one sweat session at a time.

Stay tuned, because the adventure has just begun, and we're about to transform from couch potatoes into diabetes-fighting, stressbusting, powerhouse superwomen. Get ready to sweat, swear, and succeed like never before!

Chapter 5: Stress Less, Live More

Alright, my fellow warriors in the battle against diabetes, extra weight, and that pesky fight or flight syndrome, it's time to take a deep breath and tackle a formidable foe: stress. In this chapter, we're going to learn how to stress less and, in turn, live more, all while keeping our charm and occasional swearing intact. Who knew Diabetes is also a stress disorder, right?

The Not-So-Friendly Foe: Stress

Stress, my friends, is like that party crasher who shows up uninvited, spills red wine on your favorite rug, and then insists on telling you all about their vacation to the Bermuda Triangle. It's not fun, it's not welcome, and it's something we need to deal with.

Now, stress isn't just a mental game; it's a physiological showdown. When stress kicks in, our body releases a cocktail of hormones, including our favorite troublemaker, cortisol. And cortisol, as we've learned, loves to mess with our blood sugar.

Stress and Diabetes: A Diabolical Duo

Let's talk about stress and diabetes tag-teaming your body. When stress hormones like cortisol are in the mix, they can cause your liver to release more glucose into your bloodstream. It's like your liver is having a sugar party, and insulin is struggling to regain control.

Stress can also make you more insulin resistant, meaning your body doesn't respond to insulin as effectively as it should. It's like insulin is knocking on the door, but nobody's answering. Blood sugar levels spike, and you're left feeling like you're on a blood sugar rollercoaster. Wtf right?

The Art of Stress Management

Now, we can't just wish stress away; it's a part of life. But we can learn to manage it better, like a pro. And when we do, not only do we reduce the impact on our blood sugar, but we also reclaim our sanity.

The Power of Mindfulness

Mindfulness is like the superhero of stress management. It's all about being present in the moment, focusing on what's happening right now, and letting go of worries about the past and future. Let that shit go. Rinse and repeat.

Try this: Take a deep breath. Feel the air fill your lungs, and as you exhale, let go of tension and stress. It sounds simple, but this practice can work wonders.

Mindfulness isn't just about meditation, though that's an excellent tool. It's also about bringing awareness to your daily activities, whether it's eating, walking, or even washing dishes. When you're fully present in these moments, it's like you're telling stress to take a hike.

Exercise: Your Stress-Busting Sidekick

Remember how we talked about exercise in the last chapter? Well, it's not just about weight loss; it's also an excellent stressbuster. When you work up a sweat, your body releases endorphins, those feel-good hormones that kick stress to the curb.

Exercise also helps you sleep better, and we all know that a good night's sleep is the ultimate stress-reducer. So, lace up those sneakers, my friends, and get ready to kick stress's sorry butt.

The Power of Laughter

Laughter, my friends, is the best medicine, especially when it comes to stress. It's like a little vacation for your soul. When you laugh, your body releases more feel-good chemicals, and stress doesn't stand a chance.

So, whether it's watching a comedy, telling jokes with friends, or laughing at your own cheesy puns, make laughter a part of your daily routine. It's like your personal stress-

The Cliffhanger: Embracing a Stress-Less Life

So, there you have it, ladies – a crash course in stress management that's going to help us stress less and live more. We've learned about the diabolical duo of stress and diabetes and how they mess with our blood sugar.

Stress busters come in many different flavors, breathing techniques such as the breathe in for seven counts, hold for 4 counts, breathe out for 8 counts works like a charm, Sanskrit mantras which I use twice a day, stretching, gentle yoga and Qi Gong and removing stressy negative people from your life. Works Miracles. Honest.
Stay tuned, because the adventure continues, and we're about to embrace a stress-less life filled with laughter, mindfulness, and the occasional colorful word. We're reclaiming our inner calm and taking charge of our health and happiness like the fierce warriors we are. Stress, you've been warned – we're coming for you!

Chapter 6: The Witty, Weight-Loss Wrap-Up

Well, well, well, ladies, we've reached the grand finale of our epic journey in "Sweat, Swear, Succeed." It's time to put a charming, witty, and slightly swearing bow on this adventure as we sum up our battle against the diabetes, weight, and stress trifecta. But fear not; this is just the beginning of the rest of your amazing, healthy life.

A Toast to Our Triumphs

Before we dive into our final chapter, let's raise a glass, metaphorical or real, to all the triumphs, big and small, that you've accomplished on this journey. You've battled the blood sugar dragons, outsmarted cortisol, sweated, laughed, and learned. You're stronger, wittier, and dare I say, even more fabulous.

You've made the choice to take control of your health, and that, my friend, deserves a standing ovation. So, let's give ourselves a hearty round of applause, a pat on the back, and maybe even a celebratory dance. Because you've earned it.

The Power of Progress, Not Perfection

In this quest for better health, it's essential to remember that perfection is not the goal. Nobody has it all figured out all the time. We're all a work in progress, and that's okay. In fact, it's more than okay; it's real, it's human, and it's beautiful.

There will be days when you crush your workout, make impeccable food choices, and sail through stress like a Zen master. And then, there will be days when you hit snooze on your alarm, indulge in a treat, and even drop an F-bomb or two. It's all part of the journey.

The key is to keep moving forward, to keep learning, and to keep striving for your best self. Progress, no matter how small, is still progress. It's the steps you take on the path to your goals that matter most.

Reveling in the Successes

Now, let's take a moment to bask in the successes of your journey. Have you noticed that your blood sugar levels are more stable? That you've shed a few pounds (or more)? That you're handling stress like a pro? These are your victories, and you've earned every single one of them.

Think about all the delicious, nutritious meals you've prepared, the workouts you've conquered, and the moments of laughter and mindfulness you've embraced. These are the building blocks of a healthier, happier you.

Setting S.M.A.R.T. Goals

As we wrap up this adventure, it's time to look ahead and set some S.M.A.R.T. goals – Specific, Measurable, Achievable, Relevant, and Time-bound. These are the goals that will keep you motivated and moving forward.

It's committing to a certain number of workouts each week or trying out a new recipe every month. It's aiming for a specific weight loss target or mastering a stress-busting technique. Whatever it is, make it clear, trackable, and attainable.

Remember, it's not just about the destination; it's about the journey. And the journey should be enjoyable, filled with self-discovery, and, yes, the occasional swear word.

The Power of Community

Throughout this adventure, you've had the support of your fellow warriors – women who, like you, are facing the challenges of diabetes, weight loss, and stress head-on. Never underestimate the power of community.

We've laughed, we've sweated, and we've learned together. Lean on this community whenever you need encouragement, advice, or just a virtual shoulder to lean on. You're never alone in this journey.

Embracing a New Beginning

As we come to the end of our journey, remember that this is just the beginning of a new, healthier chapter in your life. You have the tools, the knowledge, and the resilience to face whatever challenges come your way.

Embrace each day as an opportunity to make choices that align with your health and happiness. You've got the wit, the charm, and the determination to succeed, no matter what life throws at you.

The Witty, Weight-Loss Wrap-Up

In closing, my fierce warriors, I want to leave you with this: you have the power to shape your destiny, to overcome obstacles, and to create a life that's vibrant, healthy, and full of laughter. Embrace your strength, your charm, and, yes, the occasional swear word as you.

The end. But not for you dear readers. Carry on and thrive. Trust the fucking process.